How to Naturally Prevent Premature Deaths through Diet & Exercise

How to Naturally Prevent Premature Deaths through Diet & Exercise

Commission for Research and Enlightenment Book One

Daniel Dalton

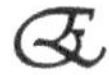

Strategic Book Publishing and Rights Co.

Strategic Book Publishing & Rights Co., LLC
USA | Singapore
www.sbpra.net

For information about special discounts for bulk purchases, please contact Strategic Book Publishing and Rights Co. Special Sales, at bookorder@sbpra.net.

ISBN: 978-1-68235-506-0

To my children, grandchildren, and readers, I encourage you to PLEASE eat sensibly and exercise regularly to avoid being overweight and obese.

TABLE OF CONTENTS

Appendix

Acknowledgements

To begin with, I wish to express my sincere thanks and appreciation to God Almighty, who inspired, instructed, and guided me throughout the research and writing of part one and two of book one under the series *Commission for Research and Enlightenment*, to Him belongs the PRAISE.

As you know, writing is a talent that a very few are born with and a craft that take years of experience to learn.

While I would like to take full credit for this book, it would be foolish of me if I do not recognize those who supported me, directly or indirectly, during the writing of the manuscript.

I wish to express my sincere thanks and appreciation to my mentors whose books and other materials, through the internet, assisted me in the development and writing of the manuscript.

1. AuthorHouse UK, for providing notes and guidelines such as "Writing Effective Dialogue," "The Importance

of Good Editing," and "Formatting Your Manuscript for Submission," and the like. These materials continue to serve as guideposts in my writings.

2. Pete Masterson, consultant, Aeonix Publishing Group, USA, who taught me about publishing and the different kinds of publishers. His notes and articles opened my eyes in understanding the mechanics of publishing.
3. Dr. Michael T. Murray, ND
4. Dr. Dean Ornish, MD
5. Dr. Peter O. Kwitterovich Jr., MD

Besides your Holy Scriptures, if you're a God-fearing person, I encourage you to buy and read the books of the three great American scientists mentioned above (see Selected References). By so doing, you'll be guided on diet and heath for natural healing, rejuvenation, and longevity.

I am also grateful to my daughter, Abigail Dalton, who provided two useful pieces of information from her phone: a video on how to burn fat, and a photo of a man with severe abdominal fat.

I also do not want to forget Matthew G. Marweah, information technology specialist, who helped to design the book cover.

Introduction

As an overweight and obese person, have you ever considered combining sensible eating with regular exercise? Do you know that diet and obesity contribute to heart disease, cancer, strokes, diabetes, and virtually every other major disease afflicting our society? Do you know that you are what you eat?

The reason why most people accumulate excessive body fat is because they take in more food energy than they spend. That is to say that they become overweight and obese because they eat more, for example, starchy foods, sugar and other concentrated sweeteners, corn syrup, and alcoholic beverages, to name a few, without exercising to burn some of the calories these foods contain.

In this book, our focus is on acquired fatness due to poor eating habits and lack of exercise, which leads to the enlargement of vital organs like the heart, liver, and stomach.

What is sensible eating? Sensible eating has to do with eating a wholesome or healthy diet. In the words of Dr. Michael T. Murray, ND, a "healthy diet is one that (1) is rich in whole, natural foods, such as fruits, vegetables, grains, beans, seeds, nuts; (2) is low in fats and refined sugars; and (3) contains adequate, but not excessive amounts of protein."

Some people are overweight because of the kind of exercise they are doing, like weightlifting for body building. Other causes are pregnancy, congestive heart failure, and nephrotic syndrome that causes the accumulation of excess body fluid, to name few. These conditions are reversible. Also, women with large buttocks and thighs can also be overweight because of the fat distribution and concentration, especially where their weight doesn't match with their height—for example, a woman who weighs 160 pounds but is only five feet tall. This doesn't match because her body mass index is above thirty (obese). At five feet tall, her ideal weight should be 95 to 100 lbs. However, this kind of fat, because of its location, is not troubling. Therefore, our focus shall be on overweight and obesity due to the accumulation of fat in the abdominal region, a predisposing factor to numerous health problems.

Do you know that the body has the mechanism to convert high caloric or starchy foods and alcohol to sugar? When these foods, like others of the same family (simple carbohydrates), are converted to sugar, "the body absorbed them rapidly, causing blood sugar to rapidly increase. When too much sugar calories enters the blood stream, the sugar stimulates the pancreas to produce insulin which increases the conversion of the sugar calories into body fat."

Other foods you should be careful with because they are high in sugar are cakes, candies, frozen yogurt, soda, flavored coffee drinks, sweet tea, and other sweet beverages like fruit juice. These foods are considered to be belly-fat givers in disguise. So, eating and drinking too much of these foods increases your chances of developing abdominal fat or belly fat.

The reason why alcohol is implicated is because it is converted into sugar and, above all, suppresses the burning of belly fat. So, you see, it has two roles to play: firstly, when converted to sugar, it helps build up body fat, and worst of all, it suppresses the burning of fat it helps to create. Notice that most people who drink beer frequently and excessively have large abdomens (belly fat) that makes them appear like pregnant women and shapeless. Despite this discouraging news about beer, when drank in moderation coupled by regular exercise, it makes your skin beautiful, reduces your risk of heart disease, keeps your kidneys healthy, and reduces your level of the bad cholesterol (LDL), to mention its few health benefits and medicinal properties. In my planned book, *Religion, Beer, and Wine,* we shall talk about the health benefits and medicinal properties of beer and wine based on scientific evidence and their use and warnings in science and the Holy Scriptures.

Why write about excess weight and obesity? Two of my very close friends died of heart failure due to hypertension and diabetes, according to the medical reports. They were from an economically balanced family with tremendous appetite for all kinds of food and drinks. They accumulated pounds of extra fat due to their poor choice of food and lack of exercise. It was their deaths that moved me to conduct the research and write the part one with the title *Suicide Bombers: Overweight and Obesity*. They indeed committed suicide and died prematurely.

As you read part one and part two, I encourage you to take the information seriously and put into practice the practical messages so that you can experience natural healing, rejuvenation, and longevity.

Part One

Suicide Bombers –
Overweight and Obesity

Well go ahead and eat and grow fat, become ugly, heavy, have asthmatic attacks and die choked. —

Brillat-Savarin (famed French gourmet)

Your chances of staying healthy or becoming healthier, of avoiding a heart attack and many other serious ailments, of living a longer, more vigorous lifetime, are increased enormously when you melt away layers and pockets of fat that burden your organs.

—Dr. Irwin M. Stillman

Do you know your height and weight? Do you know whether your weight matches with your height? Most people don't know and don't care to know. All they know, whether they are overweight or not, is that life must go on. In Africa, being overweight means that you are enjoying life; conversely, when you are underweight, people assume that you are not enjoying life, perhaps because of poverty coupled by a lack of a nutritionally balanced diet. Today, you find some African men and women with enlarged abdomens (in higher positions) working in governments. Teasingly, some people say it is the taxpayer's money that causes their abdomens to be enlarged. Are their abdomens a bank? I wonder!

What is Obesity?

Obesity means that you have an unhealthy amount of undesirable body fat. As you know, everyone needs some body fat, but too much fat can cause health problems. Obesity is a chronic, incurable, easily diagnosed, very common (epidemic) disease that is associated with life- threatening morbidity and mortality. Body fat in excess of 22 percent for young men and 32 percent for young women (the levels vary slightly with age) poses health risks. Central obesity, in which excess fat is distributed around the trunk of the body, presents greater health risks than excess fat distributed on the lower body.

According to statistics, overweight people usually die at a young age. And depending on how much excess fat you carry, you will shorten your life by one, ten, or even more years. Overweight people are cut down before their life expectancy by heart disease, strokes, emphysema (shortness of breath, difficulty in breathing), diabetes, and many other afflictions. The following death chart is based on a number of expert estimates. Some are higher, while some are lower, but these figures are generally agreed upon:

    10% overweight -------------- 10% shorter life span
    20% overweight -------------- 20% shorter life span
    30% overweight -------------- 30% shorter life span
    40% overweight -------------- 40% shorter life span
    50% overweight -------------- 50% shorter life span

In order words, if you are 10 percent overweight, your chances of dying earlier than your life expectancy are 10 percent higher. That is to say, if your ideal weight is 160 pounds and your normal life expectancy is age 70, you are likely to die at age 63. You will lose seven years of life. In effect, you will have committed suicide at age 63. This means that if you are 10 percent heavier or more than your ideal weight, then you should consider yourself overweight, taking years off your life. Looking at it another way, you are making yourself look and feel years older than you really are. Besides, you make yourself shapeless and ugly. A few extra pounds could be the difference between good and bad health. In some cases, you are actually killing yourself by staying fat. Your organs are aging and enlarged. See the illustrations below as extracted from *The Doctor's Quick Weight Loss Diet* by Dr. Irvin M Stillman:

(Female) Excess Fat Spurs Body Malformation

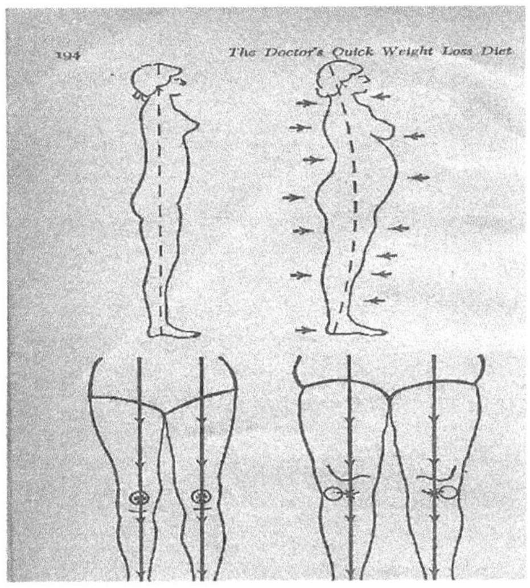

Notice how an ideal weight figure (left) is actually bent out of shape by excess weight (right), straining the muscles, body structure, and organs at many points.

In the bottom part of the illustration, notice how the weight of the body normally bisects the kneecaps and falls between the large toe and second toe. Being excessively overweight (right illustration) usually throws the feet outward. Weight does not fall at midline as desirable but beyond the kneecap and toward the back of the arch. This may produce severe osteoarthritis (bone arthritis) of the pelvis, knee, and ankle joints, with severe flat feet, varicose veins, and general fatigue.

The following illustration, according to Dr. Stillman, happens in a man 5'6" tall, weighing 190 pounds instead of his ideal weight of 130-143.

The Inside Story of Overweight Effect on Organs

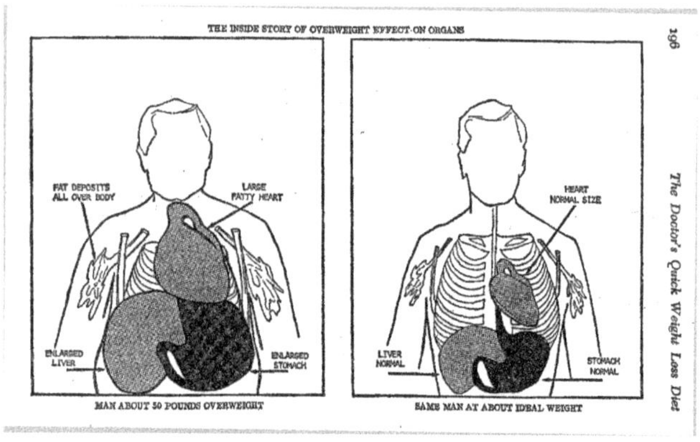

Notice that the head and neck are enlarged due to fat deposits under scalp skin and muscle layers. Fat deposits all over the body demand increased blood pumped by the heart. The heart is covered with a layer of fat, especially at the top. This is very burdensome to its proper functioning. The heart is pushed up into the neck and also brought forward. If you place your fingers between your two collar bones, you will feel distinct pulsation normally not apparent. The main blood vessels are enlarged in order to carry blood to the excessive amount of fat deposited in the arms and chest wall.

Lung capacity is reduced at least one-third because of crowding by fat. The liver is enlarged to one and a half times its normal size and is pushed up into the lung cage. The stomach is ballooned up to three times its normal size and pushes up into the chest. The abdomen is raised high because of the tremendous amount of fat in the abdominal cavity (a very large tumor or a pregnancy acts similarly).

The coronary blood vessels cannot enlarge, yet they must carry the same amount of blood to the heart muscle. If the rate of flow is increased by extra work, emotion, or a huge meal, the heart cries out that the heart muscles are being undernourished because of scant supplies of available blood. In the picture at the right, note that there is plenty of breathing space and the heart does not reach up into the neck as it does at the left.

Even small increases in weight lower your life expectancy. If you are 5 percent heavier than your ideal weight, you are not fat. But for health's sake, as well as improved appearance, you're much better off losing the few extra pounds and maintaining your ideal weight or slightly under. If you weigh 10 to 15 percent more than your desirable weight, you are obese. If you are supposed to weigh in around 130 or 140 pounds and you are pushing to 160 pounds, you are one of them—Bessie or Billy Bunter. To gain a few extra pounds and do nothing about it means you are killing yourself (committing suicide).

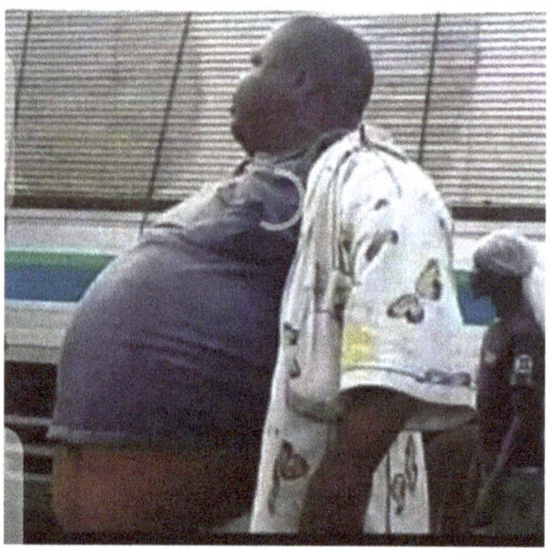

The photo is culled from Abigail Dalton's (my daughter) mobile phone Facebook page, who reported it and transferred it to my cellphone.

As you already know, abdominal fat is common in men, and at times it can be severe, as you see on this young man. Notice the entire upper region of his body is apple-like because of the excessive deposits of fat in his stomach, liver, and heart. You could hardly see his neck because the heart is pushed up into the neck and also brought forward. You can imagine what his waist circumference would be. He is a candidate for all the debilitating conditions associated with obesity. His condition is suicidal.

Overweight people are more susceptible to many common and even minor diseases. They have less resistance to infections and are far more afflicted with worse and long-lasting colds than those at ideal weight. For those carrying excess layers of fat, surgery is far more hazardous, and the anesthetist is more concerned when preparing a fat person for surgery. According to Dr. Irwin M. Stillman, any surgeon performing surgery on a fat person must worry as he/she cuts through pounds and layers of fat.

Waist Circumference

A person's waist circumference is the most practical indicator of fat distribution and abdominal fat. In general, women with a waist circumference of greater than *35 inches (88 centimeters)* and a man with a waist circumference of greater than *40 inches (102 centimeters)* have a high risk of central-obesity-related health problems such as diabetes and cardiovascular disease.

The distribution of fat on the body may be more critical than the total amount of fat alone. *Intra-abdominal fat* that is stored around the organs of the abdomen is referred to as *central obesity* or body fat and, independently of total body fat, is associated with increased risk of heart disease, stroke, diabetes, hypertension, and some types of cancers. As you know, obese people have elevated levels of hormones that could influence the development of cancer. For example, adipose tissue is the major site of estrogen synthesis in women. Obese women have elevated levels of estrogen, and estrogen has been implicated in the development of cancers of the female reproductive system—cancers that account for half of all cancers in women.

Abdominal fat is most common in men and to some extent in women past menopause, and it is closely associated with heart disease, stroke, diabetes, hypertension, and some types of cancer. In contrast, lower-body fat is more common in women than in men and is not usually associated with chronic diseases. Popular articles sometimes call bodies with upper-body fat "apples" and those with lower-body fat, "pears." Researchers sometimes refer to upper-body fat as "android" (manlike) obesity and to lower-body fat as "gynoid" (womanlike) obesity. Even when total body fat is similar, men have more abdominal fat than women. Regardless of gender, the risks of cardiovascular disease, diabetes, and mortality are increased for those with excessive abdominal fat.

Fat around the hip and thighs, sometimes referred to as lower-body fat, is most common in women during their reproductive years and seems relatively harmless. In fact, overweight people who do not have abdominal fat are less susceptible to health problems than overweight people with abdominal fat. *Source: Understanding Normal and Clinical Nutrition*

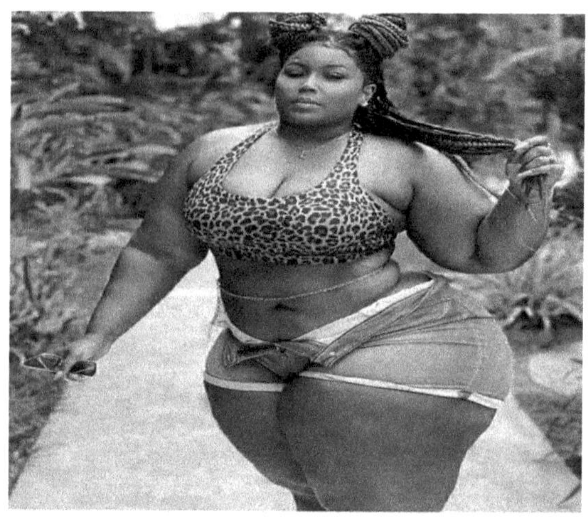

Culled from my Facebook page

This young and beautiful woman's fat is around her hips and thighs, including her arms and breast regions. Noticed, her abdomen is flat, which makes it harmless and less susceptible to health problems than overweight people with abdominal fat. Believe me, if there was a way we could check her waist circumference, it would be normal despite her being overweight. In this case, she is a healthy overweight person.

The relationship between obesity and cardiovascular disease risk is strong, with links to both elevated blood cholesterol and hypertension. Central obesity may raise the risk of heart attack and stroke as much as the three leading risk factors (high LDL cholesterol, hypertension, and smoking) do. In addition to body fat and its distribution, weight gain also increases the risk of cardiovascular disease. Weight loss, on the other hand, can effectively lower both blood cholesterol and blood pressure in obese people. Of course, lean and normal-weight people may also have high blood cholesterol and high blood pressure, and these factors are just as dangerous in lean people as in obese people. (Source: *Understanding Normal and Clinical Nutrition*)

The ideal amount of body fat varies from person to person, but researchers have found that body fat in excess of 22 percent for young men and 32 percent for young women (the levels rise slightly with age) poses health risks. Central obesity, in which excess fat is distributed around the trunk of the body, presents greater health risks than excess fat distributed on the lower body. (Source: *Understanding Normal and Clinical Nutrition*)

Weight for Height

On the following chart, the lower figure is the "ideal weight" (which may be called "desirable weight"). The higher figure is the average weight for height. These figures are for men and women aged twenty-five and over, naked or in stocking feet and without jacket or coat suit.

WOMEN aged 25 or over: 5 feet – 100 pounds. For every inch above five feet, add five pounds per inch for average weight; from that figure, subtract about 10 percent for ideal weight. The figures give you the range between ideal and average weight as a guide. For 18 to 25 years of age, subtract one pound for each year under 25. For example, a girl of 19, 5'4" tall, ideal weight = 102 pounds, average weight = 114 pounds.

MEN aged 25 or over: 5 feet – 110 pounds. For each inch over five feet, add 5.5 pounds per inch for average weight; from that figure, subtract about 10 percent for ideal weight. The figures give you the range between ideal and average weight as a guide. For 18 to 25 years of age, subtract one pound from each year under 25. For example, a young man of 21, 5'10" tall, ideal weight = 146 pounds, average weight = 161 pounds.

Height	Weight for Women	Weight for Men
5'0"	95-100	105-110
5'1"	95-105	105-115
5'2"	100-110	110-121
5'3"	103-115	113-126
5'4"	108-120	120-132
5'5"	112-125	123-137
5'6"	117-130	130-143
5'7"	121-135	133-140
5'8"	124-140	140-154
5'9"	130-145	143-159
5'10"	135-150	150-165
5'11"	140-155	153-170
6'0"	144-160	160-176
6'1"	143-165	163-181
6'2"	153-170	170-187

Source: *The Doctor's Quick Weight Loss Diet* by Dr. Stillman

Body Mass Index

Overweight and obesity are defined using a tool called *body mass index* (BMI). BMI is a way of estimating total body fat for most people. The easiest way to find your BMI is to use the table below for adults aged twenty years and older. The body mass index (BMI) is a quick and easy measure of overweight and obesity. As such, the BMI is an important vital sign that should be routinely assessed, as is blood pressure. However, the BMI is not accurate in patients with heart failure, pregnant women, and body builders. By BMI standard, overweight is different from overly fat. A BMI of 25 for adults represents a healthy target either for overweight people to achieve or for others to not exceed. Obesity-related diseases and increased mortality become evident beyond this upper limit. A BMI below 17 is a sign of illness and can result in reduced work capacity and poor reproductive function. The BMI describes relative weight and height as follows:

- Underweight falls below 18.5
- Healthy weight falls between a BMI of 18.5 and 24.9
- Overweight is above 25
- Obese is above 30

To know your BMI, do your height and weight and check for your BMI at the top on the chart. For example, my height is five feet four inches, and my weight is 154 pounds. Notice that my weight is between 151 and 157 pounds. If you check the BMI, at the top, you notice I am within the 26 range. For my height, I am overweight. Even though I am overweight, I don't have abdominal fat because I eat sensibly and expand between 1,200 to 2,000 calories weekly through brisk walking. This depends on the duration and frequency.

BMI	25	26	27	28	29	30	31	32	33	34	35	40
Ht.	Weight in Pounds											
4'10	119	124	129	134	138	143	149	153	158	163	167	191
4'11	124	128	133	138	143	148	154	158	164	169	173	198
5'	128	133	138	143	148	153	159	164	169	175	179	204
5'1	132	137	143	148	153	158	165	169	175	180	185	211
5'2	136	142	147	153	158	164	170	175	181	186	191	218
5'3	141	146	152	158	163	169	175	181	187	192	197	225
5'4	145	151	157	163	169	174	181	187	193	199	204	232
5'5	150	156	162	168	174	180	187	193	199	205	210	240
5'6	155	161	167	173	179	186	192	199	205	211	216	247
5'7	159	166	172	178	185	191	198	205	211	218	223	255
5'8	164	171	177	184	190	197	204	211	218	224	230	262
5'9	166	176	182	189	196	203	210	217	224	231	236	270

BMI	25	26	27	28	29	30	31	32	33	34	35	40
Ht.	Weight in Pounds											
5'10	174	181	188	195	202	207	216	223	230	237	243	278
5'11	179	186	193	200	208	215	222	230	237	244	250	286
6'	184	191	199	206	213	221	228	236	244	251	258	294
6'1	189	197	204	212	219	227	236	243	251	258	265	302
6'2	194	202	210	218	225	233	241	250	258	265	272	311
6'3	200	208	216	224	232	240	248	256	264	272	279	319

Source: *Obesity and the Metabolic Syndrome – Time to Recognize, Time to Treat*; Medical Education System, Inc., Department of Continuing Education

If your BMI is between 25 and 29.9, you are in the overweight category. If your BMI is 30 or above, you are in the obese category.

There are three classes of obesity:

- Class I obesity is a BMI of 30-34.9
- Class II obesity is a BMI of 35-39.9
- Class III obesity is a BMI of 40 and higher

In general, the higher your BMI is above 25, the greater your weight-related risks.

Remember, not all overweight and underweight people will get sick and die before their time, nor will all normal-weight people live long and healthy lives. These are *correlations*, not *causes*. For the most part, people with a BMI between 18.5 and 24.9 have relatively few health risks; risks increase as BMI falls below or rises above this range, indicating that both too little and too much fat impair health. People who are extremely underweight or extremely obese carry higher risks of early death than those whose weight falls within the acceptable range. These mortality risks decline with age.

An underweight person, especially an older adult, may be unable to preserve lean tissue during the fight against a wasting disease such as cancer or a digestive disorder, especially when the disease is accompanied by malnutrition. Without adequate nutrient and energy reserves, an underweight person will have a particularly tough battle against such medical stresses.

In fact, many people with cancer die not from the cancer itself, but from malnutrition. Underweight women develop menstrual irregularities and become infertile. Exactly how infertility develops is unclear, but contributing factors include not only body weight but restricted energy and fat intake and depleted body fat stores. Those who do conceive may give birth to unhealthy infants. An underweight woman can improve her chances of having a healthy infant by gaining weight prior to conception, during pregnancy, or both. Being underweight and significant weight loss are also associated with osteoporosis and bone fractures. (Source: *Understanding Normal and Clinical Nutrition*)

Independently of BMI, factors such as smoking habits raise health risks, and physical fitness lowers them. A man with a BMI of 22 who smokes two packs of cigarettes a day is jeopardizing his health, whereas a woman with a BMI of 32 who walks briskly for an hour a day is improving her health. (Source: *Understanding Normal and Clinical Nutrition*)

What are the causes of being overweight or obese?

The main creauses of being overweight or obese is eating too much and/or not being active enough. If you eat more calories than your body burns up, the extra calories are stored as fat. Everyone has some stored fat. Too much fat results in being overweight or obese. Other factors that may affect your weight include your genes (obesity tends to run in families), your metabolism (how your body processes food), your racial/ethnic group, and your age. Sometimes an illness or medicine can contribute to weight gain. (Source: National Women's Health Information Center)

For example, an adult suffering from congestive heart failure will also have generalized swelling due to the excess of fluid in the body tissues. Once, I treated a patient with 900 mg of Septrin two times daily, which was to have been used for five days. Two days after the patient was brought to the clinic, I thought my eyes were playing tricks on me when I looked at the patient, whom I hardly recognized. Her entire body was swollen. The swelling, apparently, was caused by a reaction to the Septrin tablets. Depo-Provera, a reproductive health drug to prevent pregnancy, is another potential problem I have heard about in clinical medicine. Most females gain weight when injected with the drug. These are few examples of how some illnesses and some medicines can cause someone to become overweight. Notwithstanding, this kind of overweight condition is easily handled when the condition is reversed or the drug is discontinued.

Some Serious Health Problems
Linked to Obesity

If you are overweight or obese, you are more likely to develop health problems such as heart disease, diabetes, and some types of cancer. The good news is that losing weight can improve how your heart works, lower your blood pressure, improve your cholesterol level, and lower your chances of getting other health problems.

Overweight and obesity are linked to:

1. *Heart disease*: Heart disease is one of the leading causes of death for both men and women in the United States. (It is now becoming common in Africa, especially in urban areas, according to the WHO). Heart disease includes heart attacks, heart failure, and angina (chest pain caused by reduced blood flow to the heart).
2. *Stroke:* A stroke is sometimes called a "brain attack." Most strokes are cause by a blood clot blocking an artery that takes blood to the brain.

3. *Diabetes:* Overweight people are twice as likely to develop type 2 diabetes as people who are not overweight. Type 2 diabetes reduces your body's ability to control your blood sugar. It is a major cause of early death, heart disease, kidney disease, stroke, and blindness. If you have type 2 diabetes, losing weight and being more physically active can help control your sugar levels. You may also be able to reduce the amount of medicine that you need.

4. *Cancer* of the gallbladder, breast, uterus, cervix, and ovaries (for women). Overweight men are at greater risks for developing cancer of the colon, rectum, and prostate.

5. *Gallstones or gallbladder disease*: Gallbladder disease and gallstones are more common if you are overweight. Your risk of disease increases as your weight increases. But weight loss itself, particularly rapid weight loss or loss of large amount of weight, can actually increase your chances of getting gallstones. Modest, slow weight loss of about one pound a week is less likely to cause gallstones.

6. *Osteoarthritis (wearing away of joints):* Osteoarthritis is a common joint disorder that most often affects the joints in your knees, hips, and lower back. Extra

weight puts extra pressure on these joints and wears away the cartilage (tissue that cushions the joints) that normally protects them. Weight loss may improve the symptoms of osteoarthritis.

7. *Gout (joint pain caused by excessive uric acid in the blood):* Gout is a joint disease caused by high levels of uric acid in the blood. Uric acid sometimes forms crystals that are deposited in the joints. Gout is more common in overweight people. If you have a history of gout, check with your doctor before trying to lose weight. Some diets may lead to an attack of gout in people who have high levels of uric acid or who have had gout before.

8. *Breathing problems, including sleep apnea (interrupted breathing during sleep):* Sleep apnea is a serious problem that causes a person to stop breathing for short periods during sleep and to snore heavily. Sleep apnea may cause daytime sleepiness and even heart failure. The risk for sleep apnea increases with higher body weights. Weight loss usually improves sleep apnea.

9. *High blood cholesterol:* High levels of total cholesterol, LDL cholesterol ("bad cholesterol"), and triglycerides (another type of fat in the blood) can lead to heart disease. Obesity is also linked to low levels of HDL cholesterol ("good cholesterol").

Weight loss can improve your cholesterol levels.

10. *High blood pressure:* High blood pressure is a major risk factor for heart disease and stroke. Obese adults are twice as likely to have high blood pressure as those who are at a healthy weight. Weight loss can lower your blood pressure.

11. *Complications of pregnancy:* Obesity increases the risks of high blood pressure and type 2 diabetes that develops during pregnancy. Obese women are more likely to have problems with labor and delivery.

12. *Irregular menstrual cycles and infertility:* Abdominal obesity is linked to polycystic ovary syndrome, a cause of infertility in women.

13. *Psychological and social effects, such as depression and discrimination:* One of the most painful aspects of obesity may be the emotional suffering it causes. American society (and others) places great emphasis on physical appearance, often equating attractiveness with slimness, especially in women. The messages, intended or not, make overweight people feel unattractive. Obese people often face prejudice or discrimination at work, school, while looking for a job, and in social situations. Feelings of rejection, shame, or depression are common. (Sources: National Women's

Health Information Center, Office on Women's Health, U.S. Department of Health and Human Services)

It is true that overweight or obese women/men face a lot of problems. Most drivers of commercial vehicles, especially cars, hesitate to take obese people. If the person is extra large, they will tell him or her to pay for two passenger's seats to avoid squeezing the other passengers.

Tips for Accepting a Healthy Body Weight:

- ✓ Value yourself and others for human attributes other than body weight. Realizing that prejudging people by weight is as harmful as prejudging them by race, religion, or gender.
- ✓ Use a positive, nonjudgmental description of your body.
- ✓ Accept positive comments from others.
- ✓ Focus on your whole self, including your intelligence, social grace, and professional and scholastic achievements.
- ✓ Accept that no magic diet exists.
- ✓ Stop dieting to lose weight. Adopt a lifestyle of healthy eating and physical activity permanently.
- ✓ Become physically active, not because it will help you get thin, but because it will make you feel good and enhance your health.

- ✓ Seek support from loved ones. Tell them of your plan for a healthy life in the body you have been given.
- ✓ Seek professional counseling, not from a weight-loss counselor, but from someone who can help you make gains in self-esteem without weight as a factor.
- ✓ Join with others to fight weight discrimination and fashion stereotypes.

(Source: *Understanding Normal and Clinical Nutrition*)

Part Two

Walking – The Miracle Healer

Introduction

Why did I write "Walking – The Miracle Healer"? I wrote this section because I wanted to share the experiences I've had and continue to have with brisk walking, not only as an exercise, but also as a natural healer and rejuvenator, which could subsequently result to longevity. In numbers, I'm in my mid-sixties at the time of completing this book. Physically, I feel like a healthy forty-five- to fifty-year-old man. This means I've reversed my age by fifteen years. I feel this way because of the kind of activities I'm engaged in.

I also wrote the book to share some evidenced-based scientific facts that could open the eyes and minds of those who are ignorant of the benefits one acquires when the body is regularly put in active motion through aerobic exercises.

Do you know, with the right diet and regular exercise, the body can prevent and reverse the development of debilitating diseases like high blood pressure, diabetes (acquired and inherited), heart attack, and stroke, to name a few? These diseases, according to research by the World Health

Organization, account for a quarter of the total number of deaths each year worldwide, taking an estimated twelve million lives annually. As you know, hypertension, or high blood pressure, is the commonest cardiovascular disease in most countries. It causes a narrowing of arteries that impedes the flow of blood, which is the precondition to a heart attack or stroke.

Do you know that walking can recondition the arteries and allow blood to flow freely? Do you also know that walking lowers the risk of developing breast cancer because it stops the excessive production of estrogen in your blood stream? Do you know that regular exercise, especially brisk walking, can control and/or heal high blood pressure, joint and back pain, and erectile dysfunction if done intensively with a considerable duration and frequency? I also want you to know that you seldom get sick if you do aerobic or cardio exercise regularly. Regular aerobic exercise also boosts the body's immune system.

Is exercise alone sufficient for natural healing, rejuvenation, and longevity? No, it is inadequate. Exercise without a wholesome diet and a healthy lifestyle will make you to appear like a thirsty traveler lost in the wilderness of ignorance. What we put in our body, whether in the form of food, alcoholic beverages, cigarette smoke, or narcotic drugs plays a determinantal factor in keeping our body healthy and strong or making it weak, floppy, defenseless, and possibly resulting to early death. So, exercise alone is insufficient. Be careful with what you put into your body if you want to be healthy and live long naturally. Remember, you are what you eat.

Why is good health for longevity important? Good health for longevity is important because God wants us to live as long as we're able to maintain his dwelling place (the body) properly. Without the body, no human being is human. With the body, we worship God and continue his creation as co-creators. Only a healthy body and a healthy mind can perform miracles like the creation of airplanes, computers and the internet, and cell phones, to name a few. In 3 John 2, we read: "Dear friend, I pray that you may enjoy good health and that all may go well with you, even as your soul is getting along well."

There is a common saying that those who have life have hope—that is, as long as you are alive, you should be hopeful. However, remember that faith and hope without work is dead. Do you know that a living house servant is better than his dead master, a multi-millionaire? In Ecclesiastes 9:4, we read: "Anyone who is among the living has hope—even a living dog is better off than a dead lion."

Sometimes when some people die, I hear others say that it is the person's time to die. In another quarter, they'll say it is God's time for the person to die, that it is God who has taken the person's life. I wonder why some of us continue to blame God for premature deaths, when God said we should choose between what is good and what is evil.

For example, if one chooses to drink alcoholic beverages every day in excess and damages his liver, pancreas, and heart and later dies, is it God that killed the person? If a man with a sixty-thousand-dollar vehicle stops at an entertainment center after work and consumes bottles of alcoholic beverages, gets drunk, and with blurred vision and a misguided mind drives at a speed of eighty to a hundred miles per hour, loses control on a curve, somersaults and dies, would you say it was his time to die? One of my beloved musicians, the late Michael Jackson, who I understand died after overdosing himself with his usual stuff, would you say it was time for him to die? Ecclesiastes 7:17 says: "Do not be over wicked, and do not be a fool—*why die before your time?*"

So, you see, the care of the body—in fact, your whole self (body, spirit, and soul)—is important in the sight of he who created your being. The Creator expects you to take care of your whole self—the body is no exception—in which he is supposed to dwell. Therefore, it must be properly maintained. As you know, our forefathers walked extensively and ate wholesome diets. By so doing, they experienced natural healing, rejuvenation, and longevity. In the words of Dr. Michael T. Murray, we read:

> . . . physical fitness, not calcium intake, is the major determinant of bone density. One hour of moderate activity three times a week has been shown to prevent bone loss. In fact, this type of exercise has actually been shown to increase the bone mass in postmenopausal women. ***Walking is probably the best exercise to***

start with. In contrast to exercise, immobility doubles the rate of calcium excretion, resulting in an increased likelihood of developing osteoporosis.

The Appendix covers interesting topics on sexual intercourse, compiled mainly to educate and enlighten your mind. Remember, sexual intercourse is also another form of exercise. I pray that God Almighty opens your mind so that you will understand every word and paragraph in the book; above all, practice what you learn. Remember to check your smart phone to define words you do not understand. God bless you.

Why Walk?

A walker loses weight, loses cholesterol, reduces conditions associated with hypertension, slows aging and the decline of aerobic capacity, increases strength, flexibility, and balance, strengthens bones and increases stamina. In addition, in the case of family history of diabetes, walking may help to prevent the disease.

—World Health Organization

Walking may be one of the most powerful "medicines" available. It can help lower your risk of heart disease, cancer, and diabetes, lower blood pressure and cholesterol levels, and even keep your memory sharp.

—Harvard Medical School

The third American president, Thomas Jefferson (a walker), once said: "Walking is the best possible exercise. Habituate yourself to walk very far." From my experience, as a regular walker, walking indeed is the best possible exercise because it is holistically therapeutic.

How much time do I have to exercise when I have so much to do every day? I leave my house every morning between six and seven for work and work eight to ten hours. After work, I stop at a bar or nightclub with my friends and drink a few bottles of alcoholic beverages before going home at about eight p.m. I then eat, watch TV, or go to bed. Besides that, what will I benefit from exercising when in fact some exercises are so strenuous and painful? The last time I attempted to walk just for thirty minutes, I suffered a great amount of joint pain. At between forty-five and sixty years old, I am too old to exercise, because exercise is for young people. I don't want to bother myself. I'm already suffering from high blood pressure and joint pain. I don't want my heart to beat faster than normal and cause the pressure to increase and possibly make me faint. As for the joint pain, that too could increase, so why bother myself?

The above-mentioned statements are a few among many I sometimes hear from friends and associates whenever I try to encourage them to join me in training. They make such statements because they are ignorant as to what exercise really means and the benefits thereof. I also noticed that some people who exercise on weekends do it for socialization. That is, after exercising for thirty minutes or an hour, they go to a nearby entertainment center to drink alcoholic beverages, instead of eating a banana or mango, or drinking tropical juice (mixed fruits) or water to replace the potassium, sodium, and the like after exercises like walking, jogging, and running that causes one to sweat profusely. The amount of potassium lost in sweat can be quite significant, especially if the exercise is prolonged and intensive in warm environment. That is why one feels weak and sleepy after such exercise.

I hope this discourse will serve as an eye-opener to those who think exercise is just for socialization. It is intended for those who think they are too old to exercise, and also to help those who have developed cardiovascular diseases and other debilitating conditions or are at risk of developing them.

Why is it important to exercise? According to Dr. Peter O. Kwitterovich, exercise is important for the following reasons:

1. It makes us feel better physically and mentally.
2. It gives a feeling of accomplishment and discipline.
3. It helps with weight control.
4. It generally improves one's health.

One beautiful young lady in her article captioned, "Men, if you want ladies to chase you around, here are four things you must do." Among the four things she mentioned was regular exercise. This is what she said: "Over the years, ladies have grown to love guys that exercise and keep fit. Exercise regularly, that might be what you have to do for that lady to fall for you."

Author's Testimony

Walking has become a hobby in my life. Before I started walking as an exercise, I was 160 pounds and hypertensive. Besides that, I was suffering from arthritis of the knees, fingers, and wrist. I also experienced both right- and left-upper-quadrant pains, and a lower back pain that would not permit me to have sexual intercourse. I could hardly walk well or squat. I suffered from sexual dysfunction for several months. I was five feet four inches in height and fifty-eight years old at the time. My abdomen was enlarged mainly due to club beer (Liberian made), which I drank frequently as an appetizer before eating, especially rice. My height and weight were not balanced as a result of the undesirable fat. My BMI was 28-plus. As for my right hand, it was so painful that I could hardly lift it up, and at night it became very painful. One night, I sweated profusely and my heartbeat increased. Believe me, the fear of death overpowered me. I went into the bathroom and took a bath with cold water and drank enough water. Twice, I almost fainted on the street due to dizziness. As the problems continued, fear gripped my mind. The next day, my mind stumbled over the following conditions: Angina pectoris? Prostatitis? Rheumatoid arthritis? I then decided to go for a medical examination. First, I went to a Bioform clinic, where I was examined and received the following result:

Blood Viscosity ++
Cholesterol Crystal +
Blood fat ++
Vascular Resistance +
Myocardial Blood Demand –
Myocardial Blood Perfusion Vol. +
Myocardial Blood Oxygen Consumption +
Stroke Volume +
Left Ventricular Ejection –
Left Ventricular Effective Pump –
Coronary Artery Elasticity +
Coronary Perfusion Pressure –
Central Blood Vessel Elasticity –
Brain Blood Supply Status –

The above are results of the tests and the following were the diagnoses: prostatitis, rheumatoid arthritis, cardiac decompression, and typhoid fever. A prescription was written for me to buy the Bioform drugs. Because of the high cost of the drugs, I did not buy them. I then decided to go to another clinic to do an abdominal ultrasound and ECG. The tests were done, and the following was the results:

Liver:	Size – Normal, Parenchyma – Normal, Bile Ducts – Normal
Gall Bladder:	Size- Normal, Calculi- Absent, Wall- Normal
Pancreas:	Size – Normal, Parenchyma- Normal
Spleen:	Size – Normal, Parenchyma – Normal
Kidneys:	Size – Right Kidney – Normal, Parenchyma – Normal, Calculi – Absent
	Left Kidney – Normal, Parenchyma – Normal, Calculi – Absent
Bladder:	Full, Calculi – Absent
ECG:	Normal
Findings:	3.5 x 5.0 cm functional cyst on left lower quadrant, between left kidney and spleen.

The doctor prescribed some pain killers to be taken for two weeks. I also took medication for the typhoid fever. After one week of taking the medications, the back and joint pains did not stop.

As a minister of the Gospel, I decided to pray aggressively, asking God to intervene and heal me. As an answer to my prayer, I believed, one night I had a dream in which I saw myself walking on the sidewalk in a track suit. Two days after, the Spirit moved me, and I began walking for sixty minutes every day for one month. The back and joint pains disappeared. At that time, I had not read any literature on walking, so I suffered a lot. I did not know that as a beginner I should have started with fifteen minutes, then thirty minutes, before going for sixty minutes. The first week, whenever I went to walk, I experienced weakness, dizziness, and lightheadedness while walking. Whenever it happened, I'd inhale and exhale ten times deeply and slowly, after which time I felt relief. Stubbornly, I continued to walk until I did the sixty minutes. In thirty days, my body got adjusted, and I felt like a newborn.

In 2003, a missionary friend gave me several books, among them were *The Johns Hopkins Complete Guide to Preventing and Reversing Heart Disease*, by Peter O. Kwitterovich Jr., MD, and *Dr. Dean Ornish's Program for Reversing Heart Disease*. In 2013, something moved me to search my library, at which time I noticed the said books and immediately decided to read them. It was while reading the books that I discovered the chapters on walking. It was when I realized that walking is scientific and indeed therapeutic.

For me to stop drinking beer, it was difficult. As a result, my blood pressure could not be controlled. Whenever I drank beer, I experienced headaches, neck aches, and dizziness. And when I checked my blood pressure it was slightly higher than normal. So, I continued taking drugs regularly. Once while looking through *The Complete Book of Juicing*, by Dr. Michael T. Murray, I noticed the following advice for hypertensive patients: "… eliminate alcohol, caffeine, and tobacco use. Boost potassium levels and lower dietary sodium by avoiding prepared foods and table salt . . ."

Once I noticed the recommendation, I immediately stopped drinking beer and other alcoholic beverages. I then decided to intensify my exercise and increase the duration to 120 minutes per session instead of sixty. Within sixty days, my blood pressure became normal, and I stopped taking hypertensive drugs. What happened after three years of discipline? I was no longer on hypertensive drugs and hardly got sick because my immune system, I believe, continued to be boosted as I exercised. Sexually, I was super again, despite my age.

In 2018, I again plunged into the beer and wine bottles. After four or five years of detoxifying my body with mostly plant foods and water, I purposely decided to drink, especially beer, just to find out what would happen to the high blood pressure, which was under control. The results were troubling: severe headaches and neck aches, dizziness, stomachache, and one night more heart-attack-like symptoms. It was at that point that I decided to never again let alcohol enter my body.

In late 2019, while researching and studying phytomedicine for my book *Return to the Garden of Eden for Natural Healing, Rejuvenation and Longevity*, I discovered the phytomedical treatment (plant foods) for high blood pressure and other ailments in the DASH diet (dietary approaches to stop hypertension). For the benefit of my readers check the Internet for the dash diet.

My previous weight was 160 pounds. I usually walk two times a week for 120 minutes each session at a speed (intensity) of 80–100 steps per minute. The following is my weekly accomplishments. I encourage you to keep a record of your training program, especially in the beginning. This was few years ago.

Day	Weight	Calories expended per lb. per min.	Total calories per lb. per weight	Duration	Calories expended per session
Day 1	154 lbs.	.048	7.392	120 minutes	887.04
Day 2	154 lbs.	.048	7,392	120 minutes	887.02
				TOTAL/WEEK	1,774

Note: 154Ibs x .048 = 7.392 x 120 = 887 x 2 Days = 1,774

At the time I am completing the writing of the manuscript in 2021, my weight is 154 pounds. As of 2021, after a laboratory result showed my cholesterol at 205.5 mg/dl, I increased my walking to ninety minutes three times a week, which totals 270 minutes a week. My weekly result is 154 x .048 x 270 = 1995 calories expanded. Notice that the total calories to be expanded weekly for healthfulness is a minimum of 1,200 and a maximum of 2,000.

What prompted me to order the cholesterol test? Despite the exercise, I'd been taking 50 mg of atenolol daily to control my high blood pressure, which usually fluctuated. Despite taking the drugs regularly, the lightheadedness, heart palpitations, and dizziness did not stop. These symptoms prompted me to do both the cholesterol and sugar tests. The result for the cholesterol, as previously mentioned, was 205.5 mg/dl, and the sugar was 96.0 mg/dl. Based on the result of the cholesterol test, I began taking 10 mg of atorvastatin. While taking the tablets, I also decided to research for plant foods that contain antihypertensive phytochemicals. During the exercise, I discovered the following foods:

- Bananas
- Mangos
- Cinnamon
- Ginger
- Garlic
- Pistachios
- Virgin olive oil

After the discovery, I bought a blender and started blending the banana, mango, and cinnamon to make juice (highly concentrated). The ginger and garlic were pounded in a mortar before blending, after which time I added some water and filtered it to get the liquid. It is advisable not to mix it with too much water because you have to make the juice thick or concentrated. You'll be surprised to hear that since I started eating said fruits and vegetables in juice form, one tablespoon of extra virgin olive oil, chewed a few pistachios and stopped taking the atenolol, my pressure is now normal, and the dizziness, neck aches, heart palpitations, lightheadedness, and headaches have stopped completely. Because of this result, I realized the high blood pressure may have been caused by the high cholesterol.

After one month of eating the above-mentioned phytonutrients, I decided to repeat the cholesterol test. The result was: 152.3 mg/dl (normal). As you already know, the first result was 205.5 mg/dl (high), making a difference of 53.2 mg/dl.

One thing I want you to take note of is this: no matter how much exercise you do and how well and how regularly you do it, your diet plays a very important role in your overall health. I could have died prematurely from blockages in my heart arteries due to cholesterol, which was also aggravating the blood pressure. Believe me, there were instances when I thought I was about to die, especially when the said symptoms intensified, walking became disoriented, and I was imbalanced with weak and slightly numb legs. Thank God Almighty for opening my mind to phytochemical science, which is now performing miracles in my body. I believe I have discovered a phytochemical treatment for hypertension that I'm now trying and joyfully advising others to try. You never try, you never know.

I have also cut down on eating animal flesh. As for meat, I don't usually buy or eat it. I have been a palm oil eater as an African for years. Because of its high concentration of the bad cholesterol (which I now know) and my laboratory results, I now cook with canola oil or sunflower oil, and I eat a teaspoon or tablespoon of extra virgin olive oil every day.

On November 22, 2021, I will be sixty-six years old. To further investigate my health condition, I ordered the following tests, and the results are as follows:

- Kidney Profile: Everything was normal, except for albumin (high) and calcium (low)
- Liver Profile: Everything was normal, except for albumin (high) and calcium (low)
- PSA Qualitative Test: Positive (greater than 4 ng/ml), abnormal
- Typhoid fever: Negative
- Malaria smear: No parasite seen
- HIV 1 & 2 Ab test: Normal

Frankly speaking, I was not satisfied with the PSA qualitative result because it should state a specific number other than greater than, which could mean any number. So, I decided to see a urologist, who also said the result didn't make sense. He then decided to repeat the test, including other tests based on the complaints I presented, and a test I requested (abdominal ultrasound). The following is his written report (verbatim) after the tests:

May 27, 2021

To whom it may concern,

Re: Daniel Dalton, Male (66 years) Clinic no: 007730

The above named presented to me with mainly low back pain, non-radiating, no lower limb weakness, no sphincteric problem.

He has mild nocturia, otherwise no lower urinary tract symptoms. No hematuria.

His examination is nil of note except an enlarged benign prostate. His PSA was 8.3 ng/ml, and prostate volume of 74 mls with homogenous echotexture. Normal kidney and bladder on ultrasound and normal kidney function tests were within normal range. Lumbar-sacral X-ray shows lumbar spondylosis.

He is placed on Tamsulosin 0.4 mg for 30 days and also placed on analgesics and Tizanidine.

Thank you.

The clinic and doctor's name are not mentioned due to reasons best known to me. Take note of the first PSA test and the second one from the two clinics. The second one is specific because it gives the actual number, while the first is non-specific. I was glad when the urologist told me my prostate gland is noncancerous, because this was my major concern. One of the treatments I received, however, was very troubling (Tizanidine). The drug almost killed me. Please check the side effects on your smartphone. This drug was actually for the spondylosis (a condition marked by narrowing of the intervertebral spaces and lipping of the vertebral bodies, impinging on the nerve roots). This problem developed after a fall in the bathroom. The pains in my lower back are usually off and on.

After the near-death experience, I immediately stopped taking the drug and plunged into intensive research for a natural treatment for benign prostate hyperplasia (BPH), also called prostate gland enlargement. This is what I discovered:

Tips for Naturally Lowering PSA Levels

1. Eat more tomatoes. Tomato has an ingredient called lycopene that's known to have health benefits.
2. Chose healthy protein sources, in general, going for lean proteins, like chicken, fish, and soy or other plant-based protein, is better for overall health.
3. Take vitamin D
4. Drink green tea
5. Exercise
6. Reduce stress

I say all this to say that the care of your body is the most important thing in your life, because everything you do is for your body's sake. You build a mansion to house your body; you buy an expensive car to take your body to places; you buy expensive clothes to cover your body; you eat expensive food to nourish your body, and so on. Therefore, it is mandatory, if you are to live long, to do a yearly general physical examination to possibly uncover hidden illnesses that could cause premature death. Above all, *exercise regularly* and *eat a wholesome diet.*

In my upcoming book, *Return to the Garden of Eden for Natural Healing, Rejuvenation, and Longevity,* I hope to come up with more phytochemical treatments for common ailments.

Aerobic Exercise

The word *aerobic* literally means "with oxygen," and it derives from the Greek words *aer* (air) and *bios* (life). Aerobic could then mean inhaling air (oxygen) into life (the body). During aerobic exercise, the activities of the heart and lungs are stimulated for a time period long enough to produce beneficial changes in the body. When doing aerobic exercises like brisk walking, jogging, and running, the large muscles, especially the thigh, are use in rhythmic and dynamic movements.

The three components of aerobic exercise are:

- **Duration:** How long you exercise
- **Intensity:** How fast or hard you exercise
- **Frequency:** How often you exercise

For any aerobic exercise to be beneficial, it should be comprised of a considerable duration and sufficient intensity and frequency. It should be sufficient to expend not less than 1,200 calories every week as a minimum, and a maximum of 2,000 calories. As you know, running is more intense than jogging, and jogging more intense than walking. Therefore, the more intense the exercise, the less duration it requires. Conversely, the less intense the exercise, the more duration it'll require.

The following will determine the proper length of your workouts by a calculation of the exercise you choose.

Calories Expended by Various Types of Exercises

Activity	Calories expended per one lb. per minute	Activity	Calories expended per one lb. per minute
Aerobic dance (vigorous)	.062	Rowing (vigorous)	.097
Basketball (full court)	0.97	Running (8 mph)	.104
Bicycling (13mph)	.071	Snowshoeing (2.5 mph)	.060
Canoeing (flat water, 4 mph)	.045	Soccer (vigorous)	.097
Cross-country skiing (8 mph)	.104	Swimming (55 yd/min)	.088
Golf (carrying clubs)	.045	Table tennis (skilled)	.045
Handball (skilled, singles)	.078	Tennis (beginner)	0.2
Jogging (5 mph)	.060	Walking (4.5 mph)	0.48

Source: *The Johns Hopkins Complete Guide to Preventing and Reversing Heart Disease*

Name	Exercise	Weight	Height	Calories Expended per one lb. per minute	Exercise Duration	Calories expended per session
Musu	Brisk walking	170 lbs.	5'6	.048	60 minutes	489
Mamie	Jogging	170 lbs.	5'6	.060	45 minutes	459
Mitta	Running	170 lbs.	5'6	.104	30 minutes	530

Musu, Mamie, and Miatta are of the same weight and height. I advised them to choose an aerobic exercise of their choice to help reduce and control their weight. They are centrally or abdominally obese.

For frequency, each of them did three sessions per week. The result of calories expended per week is as follows:

- Musu: 489 x 3 sessions = 1,468
- Mamie: 459 x 3 sessions = 1,377
- Miatta: 530 x 3 sessions = 1,590

If Musu, for example, is to expend the same number of calories expended weekly by Miatta, she'll have to either increase the duration per session or increase the frequency per week. To determine the amount of calories you expend per session, multiply your weight by the calories expended per pound per minute (see above). For example: 148 lbs. x .048 (brisk walking) x 60 minutes (duration) = 426.

For an exercise to be beneficial, you must expend not less than 1,200 calories, or at best work towards 2,000 calories weekly; otherwise, the exercise will be worthless. If an examination passing grade is 70, any grade below 70 is a failure. The best students are those who scored above 85 or more. So it is with aerobic exercise; the more calories you expend weekly, the better it'll be for your body physically, physiologically, and psychologically.

Below is a list of some aerobic and anaerobic exercises:

Aerobic	Anaerobic
Walking	Sprinting
Running	Weightlifting
Jogging	Push-ups
Swimming	Sit-ups
Cycling	Hand grip
Jumping rope	
Skating	

Benefits of Aerobic Exercise vs. Anaerobic Exercise

Aerobic	Anaerobic
Needs oxygen from the atmosphere to continue to contract the muscles.	Needs no oxygen but stored energy from the body.
Benefits cardiovascular system and burns more calories.	Does not benefit cardiovascular system, ends quickly, and burns very few calories.
The amount of oxygen inhaled during exercise can be measured.	The amount of oxygen inhale during exercise cannot be measured.

Source:*The Johns Hopkins Complete Guide to Preventing and Reversing Heart Disease, by Dr. Peter O. Kwitterovich*

The following additional benefits of aerobic exercise are results of studies conducted by various scientists over many years with their clients:

- ✓ Exercise decreases risk of coronary heart disease, colon cancer, osteoporosis, and stroke.
- ✓ It appears to help in the management of diabetes, obesity, and depression.
- ✓ Exercise can reverse many of the negative physical characteristics of aging.
- ✓ It can lower the systolic and diastolic blood pressure.
- ✓ Exercise slows or reverse bone loss in middle-aged and elderly people.
- ✓ Exercise can improve self-esteem, body self-concept, family relations, memory, and concentration.
- ✓ Exercise can develop your energy, make you sleep well, and improve your sexuality, despite your age (no need for aphrodisiacs).
- ✓ Depression can be prevented or treated through exercise. Since the level of norepinephrine (a neurotransmitter) is decreased in depression, exercise increases it and help relieve the victim.
- ✓ It helps in the management of stress.
- ✓ Exercise reduces major mortality rates associated with a very modest level of physical fitness.

Source: *Health Psychology, Challenging the Biomedical Model, by Charles L. Sheridan and Sally A. Radmacher*

Good health is a requirement and a must for every human being according to scripture. In 3 John 1:2, we read: "Dear friend, I pray that you may enjoy *good health* and that all may go well with you, even as your soul is getting along well." (NIV)

Walking has become so popular that it is estimated that over sixty million North Americans have discovered its unhurried pleasures and benefits. They walk to relax, to stay healthy, and to keep weight in check.

This passage by Dr. Peter O. Kwitterovich Jr. (may his soul rest in peace) is so rich and interesting that I will not paraphrase, add, or extract any word or sentence. I will present it verbatim:

Your potential for achieving a high level of fitness is established at birth. To develop this potential, you need to engage in a regular routine of physical activity. Regular aerobic exercise will also produce the following beneficial changes for you:

1. Your VO2 will be greater, and you will be able to do greater amounts of physical work.
2. Any given level of work will feel much easier to perform, and you will be able to perform for a longer period of time.
3. You will notice a decrease in your heart rate (pulse rate) and your breathing rate for the same amount of exercise.

4. Your coronary risk profile will improve: that is, you will likely have lower blood lipid levels, lower blood pressure, and relative blood fat, but a higher blood HDL cholesterol level (see below).

5. Your body's cells will be more responsive (sensitive) to the normal effects of insulin, handling your blood sugar more efficiently.

6. You will feel and look better, producing a positive change in your attitude about yourself.

If you have arteriosclerosis, exercise may allow your compensation for the reduced flow of blood and oxygen through your coronary arteries. Your collateral circulation may be improved, and the oxygen demands of your heart muscle may be reduced by a lower heart rate, lower blood pressure, and other beneficial changes of your heart muscle that enable your heart to perform more efficiently. For example, the volume of blood that your heart pumps each time it beats will be greater, thereby decreasing the number of beats needed per minute to pump a given amount of blood. The skeletal muscles in the arms and legs of a trained person use oxygen more efficiently and impose less demand on an already compromised heart for a given amount of work.

Best of the Best

1. Walking continues to control my blood pressure, keeping me fit and healthy despite my age.
2. It has reduced and controlled my weight, increased my strength, and made me more flexible. For this reason, I can work and do domestic things tirelessly. I cook, which I love so much; I clean up the house, including the outside; and I wash my dirty clothes and the like.
3. It is inexpensive as compared to some anaerobic exercises that require registration and monthly fees. All you need are soft and well-fitting sneakers. Besides some advice and instructions in the beginning, it requires no training; you are your own teacher. Just decide to walk, and then walk.
4. It can be done consistently and throughout your life. It can be done anywhere—on the sidewalks (face coming vehicles), around your house, on your stairs, on the beach, and on playgrounds.

Naturally enough, advocates of walking state that it is superior to running because you can't use running as a regular lifetime exercise and that the body was not built for running. In addition, experience has shown that joggers beyond age forty run the risk of injuring knees, ankles, and backs. Joggers land with three or four times their body weight. By contrast, always with one foot on the ground, walkers land with only one-and-a-half times their weight, according to the WHO.

Some people say Africans don't exercise. This could be true for urban Africans, not rural dwellers who walk to their farms and back home every day. Besides that, because of the unavailability of roads and other forms of transportation, the rural dwellers walk on paths to visit friends and relatives in nearby towns and villages. Once, I walked for six hours from where I was residing to visit a friend in another town. I walked in a group, and we did it intensively because of the distance. One may not consider it as exercise because we didn't label it as such, but in reality it was. This is what African farmers in the hinterlands do every day. As a result, they reap the same benefits as those who do walking as an exercise. In fact, they benefit more because of the fresh and natural diet they eat. At the time of writing this book, a female farmer in Liberia received the Golden Image Award for being 130 years old. Even though she could no longer walk to the farm, the previous walking over the years, coupled with her lifestyle and diet, kept her strong and healthy.

Walking, we understand, was brought to light in the early 1920s as an exercise by Dr. Paul Dudley White, a Boston cardiologist and founder of the American Heart Association, who began to advocate what was then considered a revolutionary treatment for his heart patients—*daily walking*. Since then, several cardiologists and lipidologists continue to include walking in their treatment packages, especially for coronary heart disease patients. Among them are Dr. Dean Ornish, MD, founder of Preventive Medicine Research Institute, and the late Dr. Peter O. Kwitterovich Jr., MD, chief of the Lipid Research and Atherosclerosis Unit at Johns Hopkins University School of Medicine. They have written and published chapters and articles on walking.

Although cardiovascular diseases are common in the industrialized world, they are also becoming common in urban areas of developing nations, particularly among middle-class professionals, according to the WHO. African "big sharks" are no exception. The moment a poor native man becomes educated and has a well-paid job, his traditional diet of fresh, organic foods changes dramatically. Instead of buying food from the local market, where fresh and natural foods are sold, he/she goes to supermarkets where frozen meat, cheese, sausage, and other high-fat and high-cholesterol foods, including foods loaded with preservatives, are sold. They begin to consume diets rich in fats and salt. They buy cartons of beer and other alcoholic beverages and drink them daily. As a result, their body structures change. They become overweight and develop pot bellies, as though they are pregnant. When advised to exercise, they give excuses. Today, many are dying prematurely from cardiovascular and other related diseases caused by their newfound diets and lifestyles.

According to Dr. Dean Ornish and Dr. Peter O. Kwitterovich Jr., walking sixty minutes a day three times a week is the minimum requirement for expending 1,200 calories weekly. This amount of exercise is said to be enough to give most of the health benefits with the least risk of injury or death. Regular exercise of this kind will make you feel better and perhaps live longer. According to a study conducted by the Institute for Aerobics Research, it was proven that walking thirty minutes a day reduces premature death almost as much as running thirty to forty miles a week.

In a nutshell, *walking thirty minutes a day, or for an hour three times a week, and expending between 1,200–2,000 calories weekly, coupled by a wholesome diet, could be one of the best recommendations for natural healing, rejuvenation, and longevity.*

Why is walking safer than some other hardcore exercises? Moderate walking is safer because it helps to protect against sudden cardiac death (and other diseases, even cancer). This is particularly important for people who already have been diagnosed with heart disease, for whom the risks of exercising are even greater, says Dr. Ornish.

Is it right to depend wholly and solely on exercise for fitness and sustainable health? The answer is no. In fact, fitness and health are not the same. One can be fit and unhealthy. Here are few examples of some young men who were physically fit but died while exercising.

It is reported that, Tony Conigliaro, formerly a star baseball player with the Boston Red Sox, had a heart attack and remained in a coma for three weeks before he died. An autopsy showed blockages in his coronary arteries. Other reported cases of death during exercise are Jim Fixx, who died while running; Pete Maravich, a former basketball star who died at age forty while playing the game after he retired; and French athlete Jacques Bussereau died while running in the 1984 New York Marathon.

The young men mentioned above, who died at tender ages, were happy and economically balanced. They may have been eating the wrong diet and indulged in unwholesome lifestyles. That could be the reason why they died of heart attacks. I say this to say that heart attacks usually occur when a small blood clot lodges in an artery that is already significantly blocked with cholesterol and other deposits, so the blood clot is the final blow in a person who already has significant arteriosclerosis.

So, you see how important it is to eat a wholesome diet and live a wholesome lifestyle, despite the exercise you do!

Let's take for example that you are exercising to reduce your weight, while at the same time eating lot of high-cholesterol and other fatty foods, including alcohol and white sugar. Have you ever tried to fill a drum with water that has holes at the bottom? You'll be wasting your time, because every bucket of water you pure in the drum will escape through the holes. This is what happens with those who think they are exercising to reduce while at the same time eating the foods and engaging in other habits that contributed to their fatness. If you want to exercise to have a height/weight balance, use a drum without holes so that your effort doesn't become fruitless or go in vain—that is, change your diet and lifestyle.

What happens during exercise? "During exercise," according to Dr. Kwitterovich, "the oxygen uptake increases gradually over the first few minutes and then reaches a plateau. At the end of exercise, the oxygen uptake returns to the pre-exercise level but does so only gradually. This means that even after you finish exercising, you continue for a while to take up more oxygen and burn more calories." Therefore, do not sit down immediately after exercise; stand for five or ten minutes, he advised.

Tips and Hints to Remember

1. Before you engage in any aerobic exercise, especially if you are above 40 years or pregnant, consult your doctor to discuss what kind of exercise will be appropriate for you. This is necessary if you have coronary heart disease or diabetes, or are obese, or you have never done any exercise.

2. Do a blood chemistry test for total cholesterol, HDL, LDL and triglyceride, including ECG; check your blood pressure, weight, height and body mass index.

3. If you are a beginner, start by walking for 10 – 15 minutes every day for one month, then gradually 30 minutes at least four times a week. Stay at the same number of minutes for at least another one month. Remember to warm up before you start walking. Do stationary jogging, dancing or few hatha yoga exercises.

4. Wear comfortable and soft sneakers and loose-fitting clothes that are appropriate for the weather.
5. Do not drink alcoholic beverages after exercise; instead, eat bananas, cucumber, oranges and drink enough water to replace potassium and magnesium lost in sweats.

To produce a significant training effect, your exercise should be of sufficient **Duration, Intensity, and Frequency.** I recommend, if you are above 40 years of age, to see your doctor before you start any intensive exercise.

Questions and Answers on Walking

Dear reader, thank you for taking your time to read the book. Remember, reading the book is one good thing you have done. Notwithstanding, the most excellent thing you could do after reading is to practice what you've read.

I'm pleased to conclude with some questions and answers from my research desk on the benefits of walking.

What has research shown about the duration of walking?

Research has shown that people who walk for at least 5.5 miles per week are likely to live longer. Walking this much at a slow pace of two miles per hour can be enough to reduce your risk of things like heart attacks, strokes, and heart failure by 31 percent. People who walk farther got even more benefit, in case you needed some extra motivation.

What happens to women who walk thirty minutes a day?

Women who walk thirty minutes a day may cut their risk of stroke by 20 to 40 percent. Just a little can do wonders in helping your blood move through your body the way it should. Any time you can spend walking is good, but push yourself a little. Getting your heart rate up can strengthen it and lower your blood pressure.

How many steps of walking is equal to five miles?

Ten thousand steps of walking equal five miles. This is good for your overall health. If you can't quite make that, any walking you do helps. You can walk your way up slowly; use a pedometer to count your steps and try to kick it up by at least five hundred each week. For Africans, or any other group of people who do not have access to a pedometer to determine the number of steps you've walked, use a hand watch to count the number of steps per minute. Having determined the number of steps per minute, if it's too low, increase your speed to a satisfactory level and remain at that speed. For me, I usually walk 80 to 100 steps per minute for a two-hour session.

Does brisk walking count as a cardio exercise?

Yes, brisk walking is a cardio exercise because it raises your heartbeat. In this case, it has to be intense and of a considerable duration to make the heart beat faster and supply more oxygen in its chambers. Remember, oxygen is a heart food.

Is walking as good as running for your heart?
Yes, if you do enough of it.

For years, many thought that really pushing yourself—and your heart rate—was the best way to strengthen your heart. But it turns out that brisk walking is just as good in cutting down your risk of high blood pressure, high cholesterol, and diabetes, as long as you do about twice as much of it as running.

How many minutes of brisk walking should you do a week if you want to lose weight?
About three hundred minutes is recommended.

That may sound a lot, but it breaks down to less than forty-five minutes a day—a reasonable target if you are serious about shaping up. Notwithstanding, if your schedule is packed, you can burn just as many calories with fewer minutes of exercise with what is called high-intensity interval training (HIIT): twenty seconds of an energetic activity like running, followed by one minute of recovery (walking). This jumpstarts your metabolism so your body can burn more fat.

How does walking lower your risk of breast cancer?
Walking lowers your risk of breast cancer because it lowers the estrogen in your bloodstream.

Women who are active are 30 to 40 percent less likely to get breast cancer. Women and men who walk briskly or do other physical activities regularly are also much less likely than others to have colon cancer. To cut down the risk, try to walk at least thirty minutes almost every day.

Why is walking good for people who have type 2 diabetes?

Walking is good for people who have type 2 diabetes because:

- ✓ It lowers blood sugar level
- ✓ It helps you lose weight
- ✓ It helps your body use sugar

Exercise helps the hormone insulin get sugar out of your bloodstream and into cells where it can be used for energy. That can lower your risk of complications from diabetes, like nerve damage and kidney disease. A ten-minute walk after each meal is enough to do the trick.

I'm suffering from arthritis, will walking help me?

Yes, regular walking can help with arthritic pains.

Are you suffering from creaky painful knees or hip pains? If yes, you have reason to start walking. For beginners, your joint fluids move around when you start walking, and that gets oxygen and nutrients to your joints and cartilage and helps prevent friction. It also strengthens your legs and core muscles. When your muscles do more of the work, your joints hurt less. A regular walk may also help to slim down, and a thinner body means less pressure on your joints.

I'm suffering from back pains, what should I do?
Walk twenty to forty minutes two or three times a week.

Most doctors recommend physical therapy for people who have chronic back pains. While that can help, walking can be just as effective. It is free and a great stress reliever, and you can do it anytime without a referral from a doctor.

Is walking good for my bones?
Yes, walking is good for your bones because it is a weight-bearing exercise.

Activities that make you bear the weight of your own body against gravity are important because they stress your bones, and that leads them to make more cells and become more solid. Other exercises that are good for your bones include high-impact activities like jumping rope, stretching, and strength training with weights. Talk to your doctor about what's best and good for you. (Source: Dr. David Williams)

Appendix

How to Lose Belly Fat in a Week
(Fast & Naturally)

All over the world, a lot of people are unhappy with their weight. There are some people who will make the effort to lose the weight that they have gained, while others will reason out that they do not have time to do anything. Aside from the usual fat that can be seen in different parts of the body, the hardest to lose is belly fat. It does not look good, and it is often seen through the clothes that people wear. It can also be a harmful type of fat because there are some diseases and conditions that develop because of this. If you are wondering how this is possible, it is because this is the type of fat that can engulf your organs.

What if you were told that it is possible that you can lose your belly fat in a week? Would you gladly take the chance and follow the things that you should do to become successful at it? You have to remember that to make this possible, you would have to commit to long-term change, especially if you would like to keep the weight off.

How to Lose Belly Fat in a Week

Gather All the Right Facts

When you would like to lose weight, you might think that all you need is the right diet and exercise. Remember that there are different facts that you need to know first. For instance, when you are losing weight, you have to remember that you will have to reduce fat all over your body and not just your belly. If you target your belly alone, you will not gain anything.

When You Are Hungry, Eat

One of the mistakes that you might make when you are trying to lose weight is that you starve yourself. This is something that you should never do, as this will only make your body store more body fat. In order to fare better, here is what you need to do:

- Make sure that you eat breakfast, since this is the most important meal of the day. You can eat a lot during breakfast because this is where your body will get the energy that is needed all throughout the day.
- Make sure that you consume about 1,500 calories a day if you are a woman and 1,700 calories if you are a man. You can probably consume about 2,000 calories if you are on a diet, but this depends on your current weight and height.

Reduce Stress
One of the mistakes that people make is that they focus so much on dieting and exercise that they forget to think about the other facets of their life, such as the stress that they encounter at work and even in their personal lives.

- If there are stressful situations that can be avoided, try to distance yourself first from those. Sometimes, stress triggers you to eat food you would not normally eat, and that can lead to weight gain.

- If there are stressful events that cannot be avoided, what you can do instead is to make sure that you destress afterwards. You can get a massage, go to a spa, or simply breathe, because this can clear your mind and not let you think too much.

Choose an Effective Diet
There are a lot of diets that are available right now. One popular diet is the liquid diet, which a lot of people say is very effective in losing weight fast. While it is true that the effects of this type of diet can be seen immediately, it will not be an effective diet that can be continued for long periods of time. The liquid diet does not have all the right nutrients, vitamins, and minerals to ensure that people stay healthy. If you can choose a diet that is as effective and will be better in the long run, choose that.

- When choosing, look for a diet that has the food that you know that you can eat. If you choose a diet that includes food that you normally do not eat, you will continually change those items.
- Choose a diet that is proven to be safe and effective.

Check Out the Right Types of Food

With every food that you eat, there is usually something better that can take its place. For instance, if you are into eating bread, you can opt for wheat bread instead of the usual white. It is true that the taste may be different, but having an acquired taste for various food products will be better in the long run.

- Make sure that you include more fruits and vegetables in your diet. Fruits can be eaten instead of desserts that are too sweet and fattening, and vegetables can be eaten as side dishes instead of pasta. Do remember to choose the right fruits and vegetables, since their nutritional content may also be different.
- Eat more protein because protein can help you develop muscles. If you have more muscles, the chances of acquiring fat becomes slimmer.

Choose Low-Fat Dairy

There are some people who cannot live without dairy food products, so it will be hard to take them away from the system entirely. What can be done instead is to choose the right dairy food products that will be as fulfilling and yet have better nutrients and effects for the body.

- Instead of full cream milk, choose low fat milk.
- Instead of flavored and sweetened yogurt, choose plain yogurt.
- Skip butter and margarine

Choose Good Fats

You should not think that all types of fat are bad. Monosaturated fat can be good for the body, and it can be acquired from certain food products. Just remember not to consume too much, because your body needs just the right amount of fat.

- Some of the food products where you can get good fat from are avocadoes and nuts.
- If you have to choose a spread for your bread, you may want to choose peanut butter, since it is healthy and can give the right amount of sweetness that your body might crave.

Note: Common sources of monounsaturated fat are olive oil (extra virgin, preferably) and canola oil.

Choose Cardio Exercises

For losing weight, cardio exercises are the best choice. You may want to lift in order to build muscles, but those muscles will not be seen under thick layers of fat. You must lose the fat through doing various cardio exercises first.

Note: Brisk walking, jogging, running, cycling, to name few, are cardio exercises. Do brisk walking, especially if you are overweight or obese and a beginner.

- Remember to begin with easy exercises before you progress to hard ones.
- As your body gets used to the exercises that you are doing, you may want to increase the number of reps that you do so that your body is challenged more and more.
- Strength training or lifting can be done from time to time but not every day, while cardio exercises can be done every day.

With all the things that you have learned above, you will be able to lose the belly fat that bothers you. You can do this in a span of one week, but do not expect the fat to be gone immediately; it will start getting smaller first until it finally disappears with the adoption of the right lifestyle.

Ways to Increase Physical Activity

- Take the stairs, not an elevator or escalator.
- Do not use a television remote control.
- Get off the bus a step or two sooner than usual.
- Do your fetching of items such as the mail; don't ask others to do your leg work for you.

- When walking through the house, market, or department store, take the longest route to your destination.
- Choose activity outdoors as much as possible (e.g., walking, gardening, sightseeing).
- Rather than eliminate trips up the stairs, think of reasons to increase the number of trips each day.
- Use a bathroom on another floor, one as far away as possible.
- Go out for entertainment instead of sitting and watching television.
- When watching television, get up and move during commercials.
- Wash the car by hand instead of in an automatic car wash.
- When shopping, walk around the mall or store before starting your shopping.

Source: *Obesity and the Metabolic Syndrome, "Time to Recognize, Time to Treat"*

Exercise and Weight Loss

Regular exercise is a necessary component of a weight-loss program for these reasons:

1. When weight loss is achieved by dieting without exercise, a substantial portion of

the total weight loss comes from the lean tissue, primarily as water loss.

2. When exercise is included in a weight-loss program, there is usually an improvement in body composition owing to a gain in lean body weight because of an increase in body mass and a concomitant decrease in body fat.

3. Exercise helps the reduction in basal metabolic rate (BMR) that usually accompanies calories restriction alone.

4. Exercise increases the BMR for an extended period of time following the exercise session.

5. Moderate to intense exercise may have an appetite suppressant effect.

6. Those subjects who exercise during and after weight reduction are better able to maintain the weight loss than those who do not exercise.

Source: *The Complete Book of Juicing, by Dr. Michael T. Murray*

Male and Female Sexual Dysfunction

Sexuality is one of the cornerstones of human existence. It is essential to reproduction and survival of the species, it is intertwined with many aspects of social relationships, and it is a significant part of life's pleasure and meaning.

Yet, disturbances of sexual functioning are quite common.

—Benjamin B. Layeh

Do you know that sexual intercourse is an exercise in its own right and can strengthen the heart muscles, lower your blood pressure, and prevent your prostate gland from becoming cancerous? Before we read the general health benefits of frequent sexual intercourse, I deem it expedient to share and enlighten your mind on some of the problems that affects us before and during the act. We shall briefly talk about male and female sexual dysfunction and the four-stage cycle of sexual arousal. I will also share with you some of the experiences I've had over the years, personally, with female partners suffering from sexual dysfunction.

Male Sexual Dysfunction

The two major sexual dysfunctions that affect men are impotence and premature ejaculation. Impotence is referred to as the inability to obtain and maintain an erection that is sufficient to complete intercourse. Impotence falls in two categories:

Primary and Secondary Impotence

Primary impotence refers to a man who has never in his life been able to complete sexual intercourse because of the failure to get an erection. Whereas, in secondary impotence, the person presents a history of being able to have sexual intercourse but currently cannot maintain an erection. Any man who occasionally cannot perform sexually because of extreme fatigue, excessive alcohol consumption, or the like would not be classified as being impotent. However, under some situations, these "normal failures" can lead to secondary impotence if the man is overly concerned and allows this temporary condition to distress him and interfere with subsequent functioning. (Source: *Maladaptive Behavior – An Introduction to Abnormal Psychology*)

Why do men have sexual problems? According to a Chicago psychologist and therapist, fear and anxiety are the main culprits. He said if you are worried about performing, it's much more difficult to warm it up and keep it up. If you are having trouble with an erection, your anxiety breaks the mood, and you haven't got a chance in hell of getting an erection.

The problem is, he continues, you can't get an erection until you regain your self-confidence, and you can't regain your self-confidence until you get an erection. He also mentioned the "right sexual partner," who he said is someone that is willing to place higher priority on your sexual needs—and solving them—than on her immediate sexual needs, someone with whom lovemaking is a caring experience, someone who cares more about making love than having sex. (Source: *How to Make Love to a Woman*)

True story: Once, my senior medical officer, a Korean missionary doctor, and I went to a nearby nightclub in Kakata City, Liberia, to have fun. We drank enough beer, and he decided to take one of the girls we entertained home. I decided not to take home any because I was drunk. In the morning, the girl came to my apartment requesting that I tell the doctor to pay her for the night. When I went to him, I told him if he hadn't paid the girl for the night, he should do so. He argued, saying that he was not able to have sexual intercourse because he was drunk. Notwithstanding, I persuaded him to pay the girl, and he did.

From my experiences, beer or wine drank in small amounts enhance sexual arousal and performance, but when drank in excess, they can lead to secondary impotence. On the contrary, I had a girlfriend who drank up to four pints of beer or stout before sexual intercourse. And during the act, she appeared more aroused and active than when she hadn't taken any alcohol, unlike me. If I made an attempt to drink such an amount, it would result in temporary or secondary impotence.

We must remember that a penis won't perform on demand. Only sexual excitement can make a man stiff. The more you worry about an erection, the more it will smother the sexual excitement and the less likely an erection becomes. Psychologically, the best cure for impotence is to go to bed consciously rejecting the possibility of having an erection and engaging in intercourse. (Source: *How to Make Love to a Woman*)

Acupuncture, we understand, can treat primary impotence. Other traditional healers also claimed to have cures. I have successfully helped patients with secondary impotence by prescribing Energa (a

100 percent natural food supplement) and an herb: ginseng. *Please consult your doctor before you use any of the suggested remedies.* Regular exercise, however, is the best.

Premature Ejaculation

The most common ejaculatory problem in men is premature ejaculation, in which ejaculation occurs shortly after vaginal entry or even before the entry is made. Ejaculation in less than one minute was considered premature in the past. Other authorities stated that ejaculation before the female achieved orgasm on 50 percent of sexual encounters was premature. (Source: *Maladaptive Behavior – An Introduction to Abnormal Psychology*)

The second disorder in men is what is referred to as ejaculatory incompetence or retarded ejaculation, which is the opposite of premature ejaculation. Men with this problem are usually unable to ejaculate when the penis is in the vagina.

Personally, I have encountered both problems. I noticed that when I am overexcited, especially when meeting a woman for the first time, that it sometimes results in premature ejaculation. Secondly, if my partner plays with my penis for a long time, especially the glans, it will sometimes cause premature ejaculation just after entering the vagina in less than a minute.

I've also experienced ejaculatory incompetence. This usually happens when I drink a small amount of either beer or wine. During sexual intercourse, my penis will remain erect in the vagina for more than five minutes, and in some cases my partner would have achieved orgasm while I was struggling to ejaculate. In some cases, my partner would tell me to stop, especially where she had achieved orgasm and was then feeling pain. The pain, I noticed, was sometimes caused when the vagina was no longer lubricated. In this case, during the second rounds, if she agreed and was ready, I used KY Jelly to lubricate the vagina. Psychologically, it is troubling when one experiences either premature or ejaculatory incompetence, especially the latter when one fails to expel the ejaculate. It usually appears as if you've not had sexual intercourse. Ejaculation, as you already know, results in sexual satisfaction.

Female Sexual Dysfunction

There are four female sexual dysfunctions that has been identified, some are troubling while others can be easily handled with the right approach. They are as follows:

Orgasmic Dysfunction

Orgasmic dysfunction refers to the inability to achieve the orgasmic phase of the sexual response. It is primary if the woman has never achieved orgasm at all. It is secondary if she has been orgasmic in the past but cannot achieve it now. (Source: *The Psychopathology of Women*)

The major sexual dysfunction in females is orgasmic dysfunction, which refers to the inability to experience orgasm. According to the normal sequence of sexual response, the woman cannot advance beyond the plateau phase of arousal. In some ways, orgasmic dysfunction is the female counterpart of impotence. (Source: *Maladaptive Behavior – An Introduction to Abnormal Psychology*)

Situational Orgasmic Dysfunction

Situational orgasmic dysfunction is when a woman experiences an orgasm in one situation but not others; it is absolute if the woman cannot achieve orgasm in coitus or with any other kind of stimulation. Women with orgasmic dysfunction may have a strong sexual drive and be easily aroused and develop vasocongestion and lubrication but cannot reach orgasm. Some women, because of the makeup of their bodies, require prolonged, continuous stimulation of the clitoral area before they are "ready." Such women will definitely not achieve orgasm in penile-vaginal intercourse lasting for a few minutes. (Source: *The Psychopathology of Women*)

Experience shows that clitoral stimulation is very important in producing orgasm. Indirect stimulation of the clitoris normally occurs during intercourse, although more intense stimulation is possible with more finger manipulation by the woman herself or her partner. (Source: *Maladaptive Behavior – An Introduction to Abnormal Psychology*)

There is generally considerable disparity in orgasmic times between men and women. A man usually achieves orgasm in four minutes, whereas a woman needs from ten to twenty minutes of sexual intercourse before she obtains orgasm. (Source: *The Psychopathology of Women*)

Vaginismus

Vaginismus is an involuntary closing of the muscles at the entrance to the vagina, making penetration and intercourse impossible.

Dyspareunia

This refers to vaginal pains during sexual intercourse, which is sometimes caused by infection or a dry vagina (unlubricated).

Author's Experiences: Vaginismus is a problem found in some girls and women who underwent female genital mutilation or circumcision. I had three girlfriends in years past whose vaginal muscles were so constricted that penile penetration was difficult due to the manner in which the procedure was performed. According to one of the myths, it is believed that male sexual pleasure is enhanced in a smaller vaginal opening. This is in reference to the Type III classification of FGM (below right). It is also true that it could be caused by infection or a dry vagina. Besides the infection, which can be treated when diagnosed, with the other possible causes, I have successfully penetrated the vagina when I used KY Jelly or Vaseline. In some instances, I asked them to kneel and penetrated from the back.

Take note of some of the problems women experienced ignorantly because of FGM. I've had sexual intercourse with initiates whose clitoris was cut off. As a result, they hardly experienced orgasm and sexual pleasure.

Classification of FGM

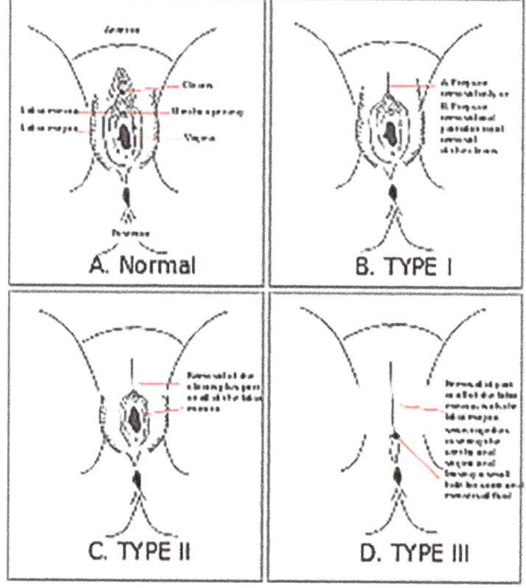

Type I: Excision of the prepuce of the clitoris with or without excision of part or the entire clitoris.

Type II: Excision of the clitoris with partial or total excision of the labia minora.

Type III: Excision of part or all of the external genitalia and stitching/narrowing of the vaginal opening (infibulation). Approximately 15 percent of women and girls who are subjected to FGM undergo this type.

(Culled from my upcoming book: *Stop Violence Against Women (Stop Beating, Raping, Killing and Circumcising Females)*

I've also had an experience with a young woman who suffered from both vaginismus and dyspareunia. Besides the pains and difficulty in penetrating the vagina, there was slight bleeding. In fact, her groaning and twisting of her body because of the pains made the act not pleasurable. Because of the pains she was experiencing, I decided to stop the act, since it was my first time having sexual intercourse with her.

From my interview, she told me that she usually experienced the pains and slight vaginal bleeding whenever she had sexual intercourse. Because of that, she avoided having sexual intercourse with men. She is a mother of one girl child over twenty years old. Since then, she has not had another child, and her relationships with men don't usually last long. Yes, it is true, because since the day she spent the night with me and I had that experience, she never visited me again. Truly speaking, would you believe that we planned to get married? What an embarrassment that could have been for me.

As a medical practitioner, I advised her to see a gynecologist to ascertain the cause of her problem. She was also suffering from pelvic inflammatory disease (PID), which I successfully treated before we had our first and only sexual intercourse. I prayed that her problem was not cervical cancer. Could it be a complication of FGM? Possibly, because she was initiated into the Sandi Society, where girls and women are circumcised.

The Four-Stage Cycle of Sexual Arousal

Excitement Phase
This phase begins with sexual stimulation of various sorts, including physical contact, sexual fantasies, visual stimuli, and so on.

Plateau Phase

This is characterized by heightened sexual arousal. If the sexual stimulation is insufficient or stopped the person will not go beyond the plateau phase. However, if there is continued intense sexual stimulation, the person progresses to phase three.

Orgasmic Phase

This is an involuntary reaction lasting for only few seconds.

Resolution Phase

This happens after an orgasm when the sexual tension drops.

The following dialogue is an interview conducted by one of the writers of the book *How to make Love to a Woman:*

> *"What are you writing about now?" she asked me with a smile.*
>
> *"Seduction and arousal," I said, a little reluctantly.*
>
> *She looked at me askance. "Is that supposed to be a hint?"*
>
> *"Only if you want it to be," I said.*
>
> *Then she said something that surprised me. "Which are you going to write about first?"*
>
> *"What do you mean?"*
>
> *"Seduction or arousal? Which one are you going to talk about first?"*

"Well, they are more or less the same thing, so I thought I'd talk about them together," I said.

The smile disappeared, and she suddenly seemed indignant. "What do you mean 'they're the same thing?' They're not the same thing at all."

I was so surprised, all I could think to say was, "I don't understand. Why are they different?"

"Arousal," she said, "is for dogs (cats). Dogs (or cats) can get aroused rubbing up and down on someone's leg. Sometimes I think men are the same way. Women get aroused, too, because we're animals. But arousal isn't enough; it's not even close. Arousal is nothing without seduction. Seduction is something extra. It's something that happens to the mind. If I'm aroused without being seduced, it's just an inconvenience, like indigestion, or the tickle that makes you sneeze."

Whatever you call them, there are really two things that have to happen before a woman is ready to make love. First, she has to *want* it. Her mind (and heart) has to be made ready for it, willing to accept it, emotionally eager for it. This part is what she refers to as "seduction" and usually happens out of bed. The second part, which may be the easier part, is physical. She has to be "primed" to make love. Her body has to be ready for it. This is what she refers to "arousal" and usually happens in bed.

I don't think the labels matter. What does matter is that helping a woman reach the stage where she is ready for lovemaking requires attention to both her emotional and her physical needs. (Source: *How to Make Love to a Woman*)

If you ask me what part of a woman's body attracts me the most, my answer would be the breasts and buttocks, seldom the thighs. As for the buttocks, not too large, but sizeable for massaging and a sizeable breast to suck and play with. I'm not attracted to obese women or very slim women.

Experience tells me that there are three parts of a woman's body that are like a magnet that has the capacity to capture the mind of most men. They are the buttocks (for most African men), the breasts, and the thighs. So, we have breast lovers, thigh lovers, and buttocks lovers.

What about women, what part of a man's body is the sexiest? Most women will say the eyes and buttocks; the hands rank third.

Women who are eye lookers uniformly believe that the eyes speak a language of their own. They believe they can read a man's whole character in his eyes. They can tell if he is gentle or strong, lustful or loving, callous or caring. According to a female doctor, "It's all in eye contact. If his eyes dart around and avoid you nervously, that's a sure sign he's not self-confident. A man who can't sustain eye contact with a woman is a washout—with me at least." (Source: *How to Make Love to a Woman*)

Remember that your eyes are the part of your body that can convey that message most convincingly, whether you are in a crowd or alone in bed.

Banana, A Sexual Intercourse Booster

Just as it is important to look after other health problems in your body, it is also of great importance that you ensure your sexual function is up to "standards."

There are many possible reasons why men lose their sex drive, and some of them include stress, depression, tiredness, too much alcohol consumption, certain medications such as hypertension drugs and anti-depressants, and above all, low testosterone levels.

Thankfully, there are certain foods that can help fire up your libido. Examples of such foods include bananas, sunflower seeds, maca, raw nuts, and celery.

Low Testosterone and Sexual Drive

Testosterone is a hormone produced by the testicles of men. It is responsible for men's sexual development and plays a role in their appearance. Testosterone is known to boost sex drive and stimulate sperm production. Due to these very important functions of testosterone, I doubt if there's anyone out there who wants his hormone level to go low. Of course, low levels translate to reduced functioning.

As a man grows older, his testosterone levels decrease. In general, testosterone production typically decreases with age. According to an American foundation, Urology Care, about 4 out of 10 men over the age of 45 have low testosterone. It is seen in about 2 out of 10 men over the age 60, and 3 out of 10 men aged 70 and beyond.

When a man's testosterone level gets low, there are numerous symptoms or signs he may experience. First of all, there is a great tendency for a reduced libido or desire to have sex. Secondly, there may be reduced erections. This is because testosterone is indirectly involved in erections, with the hormone responsible for stimulating receptors in the brain producing nitric oxide, which in turn triggers a series of chemical reactions necessary for an erection to occur.

Low testosterone levels can also cause low semen volume, fatigue, hair loss, decreased bone mass, and loss of body mass in men. But how can one curb low levels of this hormone? There are certain foods that naturally increase testosterone levels, and some these foods include garlic, pomegranates, coconuts, olive oil, and cruciferous vegetables like cabbage, broccoli, and cauliflower. Are we forgetting bananas?

Banana and Libido-Boosting Properties

Bananas have been hailed for their libido-boosting properties for a long time. Some folk healers have been recommending bananas for increased sexual function, even when there was no scientific evidence to back the claim. Perhaps it is because of their shape (looking like an erect penis). True or false?

Now there are evidence to validate banana libido-boosting effects. Bananas contain an enzyme known as bromelain, which is also found in pineapples. Bromelain has been found to increase libido. Researchers at the University of Tasmania found supplementation with just one gram of bromelain daily was enough to maintain testosterone levels in the blood. This is especially beneficial to the athletes, since extreme exertion such as running can lower testosterone levels. Apart from bromelain, bananas are a rich source of many minerals and vitamins, especially the B group. Just 100 grams of banana provides more than 20 percent of the daily requirement for vitamin B6, which has been found to boost testosterone levels both directly and indirectly.

According to Testosterone Resource, vitamin B6 promotes the production of androgens, which causes testosterone level to rise. This same vitamin has also been used to help low prolactin levels, another hormone that has been associated with unimpressive levels of testosterone.

One particular research, although carried out on laboratory animals, found those animals that were given a vitamin B6-free diet to have lower testosterone levels than those given a diet containing vitamin B6.

Moreover, bananas are a great food to improve blood circulation. Improved circulation means improved erections!

Not long ago, the flow of potassium ions in brain cells was linked to sexual arousal. Don't forget that bananas are the richest fresh fruit sources of potassium. Serotonin is believed to help regulate sexual desire and function. Bananas are not only good for sexual function, but they can also improve heart health, prevent kidney disorders, and improve digestive function.

I'll feed you with more information on bananas in my upcoming book *Return to the Garden of Eden for Natural Healing, Rejuvenation and Longevity.*

Remember to turn your phone off before you engage in sexual intercourse! Otherwise, if the phone rings, it could deflate the entire exercise …

Seven Scientific Reasons Why You Should Have Sex Everyday

1. ***It could lower his risk of prostate cancer.*** According to a study by Harvard Medical School, men who ejaculated more often reduced their risk of developing prostate cancer by 22 percent. Researchers still don't know why that is, but hey, if you needed one more reason to hit that tonight, having your guy avoid getting cancer is a pretty solid one.

2. ***Your chance of getting a cold goes way, way down.*** Researchers at Wilkes University in Pennsylvania found that people who had sex at least twice a week released more antigens like immunoglobulin A,

which helps fight off colds and the flu, so just think of how healthy you'd be if you had sex all seven days. You'd be basically immortal is what I'm trying to say.

3. ***It keeps you looking super young and confident.*** In a study by Scottish researcher and clinical neuropsychologist David Weeks, judges guessed the ages of 3,500 European and American women and men and found that the people whose age was underestimated by seven to twelve years were also reporting having sex three times a week, in comparison to the control group that was doing it twice a week. They also found these young-looking babes to be really comfortable and confident about their sexual identity. Win, win, win, win.

4. ***It'll help get rid of your heinous menstrual cramps.*** A study in 2020 found that 9 percent of 1,900 women were masturbating solely to get rid of their menstrual cramps. There's no way that many masturbating women are wrong.

5. ***It could make you crazy-fertile if you're trying to conceive.*** A new study in *Fertility and Sterility* found that having sex every day could help prepare your immune system for pregnancy, which is critical in terms of increasing your chances of having a baby.

6. ***It lowers your blood pressure and your ability to stress out over basically nothing.*** A 2005 study found that people who had penile-vaginal intercourse (their words, not mine) had lower blood pressure and better stress responses than people who didn't (or those who masturbated or had non-penetrative sex), which in theory would mean they were also way more chill. Never a bad thing.

7. ***Sex can actually make you a super genius.*** Separate studies by researchers at the University of Maryland and Konkuk University in Seoul, South Korea, found that mice and rats who had sex more often were also less stressed, and since stress makes your brain less able to function, that made them more intelligent thinkers.

So, in theory, having sex every single day would make you fertile, live longer, never get sick, and have the brain of noted genius Beyoncé. Basically, sex makes you a superhero. That's my takeaway from this.

Twelve Reasons You Should Have Sexual Intercourse Everyday

Are you stressed? Struggling to sleep? Turns out there are a number of ailments that can be cured simply by having sex regularly. Here are twelve reasons why you and your partner should be having sex daily!

1. Relieves stress

When you have sex, your body produces dopamine, endorphins, and other feel-good hormones. This makes sex an awesome stress reliever.

2. Exercise

Sex is about as good as other types of exercise. Sex for just fifteen minutes three times a week is the same as jogging for about an hour.

3. Lowers high blood pressure

Sex lowers high blood pressure and reduces diastolic blood pressure. If you're looking for something a little less romantic, hugs do the same thing.

4. It boosts your immune system

Immunoglobin A is an antigen that fights off infection, and it's increased when your frequency of sex increases.

5. You'll look younger

Having sex three times a week may help you look up to ten times younger, according to one study published in *Secrets of the Super Young*. Can't argue with that!

6. Your heart will be stronger

This ties in with exercise. If you exercise more, your heart will be stronger. All that sex is a big boost to your cardiovascular system.

7. Pain relief

Dr. George E. Elrich is an arthritis specialist from Philadelphia. He conducted a study on the link between arthritis and sex and found that those who had sex more often experienced less pain.

8. Lowered risk of cancer

Routine ejaculation in men reduces the chance of getting prostate cancer, and an Australian study found that men who ejaculated twenty-one times a month were less likely to develop the cancer.

9. Better sleep

Just like with any exercise, the increased heart rate when you have sex leads to relaxation afterward. If you're an insomniac, have some sex! It'll help you sleep.

10. Regular periods

Sex helps regulate hormones in women that makes the menstrual cycle a bit more routine. Stress is one of the biggest reasons women miss periods too. Stress relief will help make the period more routine too.

11. No erectile dysfunction

Half of men older than forty suffer from erectile dysfunction of some kind. That doesn't bode well for me! The best medicine is . . . sex! Erections help keep the blood flowering correctly and prevents erectile dysfunction.

12. You'll live longer

Summing it all up, less stress, a stronger heart, increased circulation of oxygen, and happiness are all factors that help you live longer! And who doesn't want to live a little bit longer?

Note: Remember, you never try, you never know. I hope you enjoyed reading the book.

SELECTED REFERENCES

Al Issa, Ihsan. *The Psychopathology of Women*. New Jersey: Prentice Hall, 1980.

Holy Bible, New International Version.

Kwitterovich Jr., Peter O., MD. *The Johns Hopkins Complete Guide to Preventing and Reversing Heart Disease*. Prima Health Publishing, 1998.

Lahey, Benjamin B. and Anthony R. Ciminero. *Maladaptive Behavior – An Introduction to Abnormal Psychology*. Illinois: Scott, Foresman and Company, 1980.

Medical Education System. "Obesity and the Metabolic Syndrome – Time to Recognize, Time to Treat– A Continuous Education Monograph for Physicians, Nurses and Pharmacists."

Morgenstern, Michael. *How to Make Love to a Woman*. New York: Crown Publishers, 1989.

Murray, Michael T. ND. *The Complete Book of Juicing (revised and updated)*. New York: Clarkson Potter/ Publishers, 2013.

Ornish, Dean, MD, *Dr. Dean Ornish's Program for Reversing Heart Disease*. Ballantine Books, 1996.

Rolfes, Sharon Rady; Kathryn Pinna, and Ellie Whitney. *Understanding Normal and Clinical Nutrition, Seventh Edition.* Brooks Cole, 2005.

Sheridan, Charles L., and Sally A. Radmacher. *Health Psychology – Challenging the Biomedical Model.* New York: John Wiley and Sons, Inc., 1991.

Stillman, Irwin Maxwell, MD, D-IM, and Sam Sinclair Baker. *The Doctor's Quick Loss Weight Diet.* Dell Publishing Company, May 1969.

World Health Day 1992 Information Kit. "Heartbeat, the Rhythm of Health."

About the Author

Daniel Dalton is a minister of the Gospel, a healthcare professional, and a researcher/writer in phytomedicine, health science, and religion.

He has written and published one book, *Women of Substance and Integrated*, and several articles published both locally and internationally. He was a columnist in the *Curia* newspaper, a contributing writer in the World Health Organization (WHO) quarterly newsletter, the Partnership for Health, Christian Health Association of Liberia's (CHAL) newsletter, and *Venture Inward*, a quarterly newspaper published by the Association of Research and Enlightenment in Virginia Beach, Virginia in the United States. He is a former member of the Association of Research and Enlightenment and the Charles Mason Ramey Society for Comparative Religions, both in the USA.

As a humanitarian, he founded and organized the Paradigm of Consciousness Ministries (PARACOM), which operated for ten years in the health sector in Liberia; constructed, rehabilitated, and operated clinics; constructed hand pump wells; and trained traditional midwives and skilled training for women, to name a few. In 2019, to continue his humanitarian services, he again founded and organized another NGO: Integrated Services for Humanity (HIS). The areas of intervention are in health, agriculture, and gender-based violence. He currently serves as chief executive officer of the organization.

As founder of the book series *Commission for Research and Enlightenment*, some of the planned upcoming books include:

- How to Naturally Prevent premature death through diet and exercise
- Stop Violence Against Women (Stop Killing, Beating, Raping and Circumcising Females)
- Who Killed Jesus, the Greatest Messiah
- Return to the Garden of Eden for Natural Healing, Rejuvenation, and Longevity

His hobbies include reading, writing, cooking, brisk walking, swimming, singing, and aerobic dancing.

Review Requested:

We'd like to know if you enjoyed the book.
Please consider leaving a review on the platform
from which you purchased the book.